Peyronie's Disease

A Beginner's Quick Start Overview and Guide on Managing the Condition through Nutrition, With Sample Recipes

mf

copyright © 2022 Mary Golanna

All rights reserved No part of this book may be reproduced, or stored in a retrieval system, or transmitted in any form or by any means, electronic, mechanical, photocopying, recording, or otherwise, without express written permission of the publisher.

Disclaimer

By reading this disclaimer, you are accepting the terms of the disclaimer in full. If you disagree with this disclaimer, please do not read the guide.

All of the content within this guide is provided for informational and educational purposes only, and should not be accepted as independent medical or other professional advice. The author is not a doctor, physician, nurse, mental health provider, or registered nutritionist/dietician. Therefore, using and reading this guide does not establish any form of a physician-patient relationship.

Always consult with a physician or another qualified health provider with any issues or questions you might have regarding any sort of medical condition. Do not ever disregard any qualified professional medical advice or delay seeking that advice because of anything you have read in this guide. The information in this guide is not intended to be any sort of medical advice and should not be used in lieu of any medical advice by a licensed and qualified medical professional.

The information in this guide has been compiled from a variety of known sources. However, the author cannot attest to or guarantee the accuracy of each source and thus should not be held liable for any errors or omissions.

You acknowledge that the publisher of this guide will not be held liable for any loss or damage of any kind incurred as a result of this guide or the reliance on any information provided within this guide. You acknowledge and agree that you assume all risk and responsibility for any action you undertake in response to the information in this guide.

Using this guide does not guarantee any particular result (e.g., weight loss or a cure). By reading this guide, you acknowledge that there are no guarantees to any specific outcome or results you can expect.

All product names, diet plans, or names used in this guide are for identification purposes only and are the property of their respective owners. The use of these names does not imply endorsement. All other trademarks cited herein are the property of their respective owners.

Where applicable, this guide is not intended to be a substitute for the original work of this diet plan and is, at most, a supplement to the original work for this diet plan and never a direct substitute. This guide is a personal expression of the facts of that diet plan.

Where applicable, persons shown in the cover images are stock photography models and the publisher has obtained the rights to use the images through license agreements with third-party stock image companies.

Table of Contents

Introduction	7
All About Peyronie's Disease	9
How exactly does Peyronie's Disease affect the penis?	10
Stages of Peyronie's Disease	10
Causes	11
Symptoms	12
Treatment of Peyronie's Disease	16
Alternative Treatments	17
Dealing with Peyronie's Disease	21
Schedule a doctor's appointment	21
Talk to someone you trust	22
Involve your partner	22
Remember that you are not alone	23
Create a safe space in your relationship	23
The Connection Between Diet and Peyronie's Disease	25
Implementing Your Diet Plan	27
Step 1: Decide which meal planning style suits you	27
Step 2: Stock up your pantry	27
Step 3: Incorporate your plan into your social activities	28
Step 4: Learn to read nutrition labels	29
Step 5: Get rid of certain foods and bad habits	30
Step 6: Leverage easy meal prep tips	31
Sample Recipes	33
Garlic Hummus	34
Salmon and Asparagus	35
Tahini Salmon	36
Salmon with Avocados and Brussels Sprouts	38
Chicken Breast Delight	41
Steak with Olive Oil	42

Garlic Broccoli Salad	44
Mixed Vegetable Roast with Lemon Zest	45
Spinach and Watercress Salad	46
Vegetable Broth	47
Salad Medley	49
Quinoa Lentil Salad	51
Fruit and Dark Greens Salad	53
Conclusion	**55**
References and Helpful Links	**56**

Introduction

According to statistics, at least 1 in 100 adult men in the US, or at least 10% of men aged between 50 and 60 years, develop Peyronie's Disease.

It is a condition that affects the male sex organ, causing it to bend, curve, or lose length or girth. The condition occurs when there is inflammation in the tissues of the penis, resulting in scar tissue buildup and abnormal curvature of the organ. This could be either perpendicularly or horizontally curved.

However, based on the description of the disease, it is not surprising to assume that there are probably silent sufferers of Peyronie's Disease that aren't in the statistics. It is most likely that they are embarrassed to discuss the condition with their partners, doctors, or anyone else.

There are ways to treat this disease once you get properly diagnosed with it, so do not lose hope. Aside from that, you can also try to improve your overall health by following a Peyronie's Disease Diet, which may not technically treat the disease but will be beneficial for you, especially in the long run.

In this beginner's quick start guide, you will discover:

- All you need to know about Peyronie's Disease
- Its causes and symptoms
- How to deal with it
- Treatment and procedures for the disease
- Diet for those with Peyronie's Disease

All About Peyronie's Disease

Peyronie's Disease is a condition that develops in the tissues of the penis, resulting in scar tissue buildup and abnormal curvature of it. The disease causes pain, especially when having sex or trying to get an erection.

Often, the scar forms on the top of the penis and causes it to curve upwards during an erection. If the scar is at the bottom of the penis, in that case, it will bend downwards. If the scar forms on the side, the penis curves to the side. In other cases, the scar goes around the penis, causing it to narrow like the center of an hourglass.

This disease is linked to genetics or blunt trauma to the penis, which causes the development of fibrous plaques, hardening the penis and causing the shaft of the penis to bend. As curvature worsens over time, it ultimately leads to difficult or painful intercourse; or makes it impossible altogether.

One thing to note though, some men have Peyronie's Disease but don't have the curve, and vice versa. Some men have had a curvature throughout their lives but do not have Peyronie's

Disease. The best way to know if you have this is by getting properly diagnosed by a medical professional.

How exactly does Peyronie's Disease affect the penis?

Penises have two important functions: for urination and sexual intercourse, particularly ejaculation.

Inside the penis lies three tubes: the urethra and a couple of corpora cavernosa.

- The urethra is responsible for carrying urine from the bladder through the penis.
- The two corpora cavernosa allows the penis to be erect.

During intercourse, blood flows to the penis, making it straight, stiff, and hard, ready for penetration. After an orgasm, semen leaves the urethra–a process called ejaculation. It's important to note that the disease affects the shape and size of the penis but not its functions–ejaculation or urination.

Stages of Peyronie's Disease

- **Acute phase**

    This phase is marked by the formation of softer and pliable plaques within the penis, causing it to increase in size and develop shape. It is hard to detect any symptoms during the early months of this phase, which lasts for about 6-12 months. As the plaques harden over time, the patient experiences pain and discomfort, especially during an erection.

- **Chronic phase**

    During this phase, the scar is fully formed and hardened. This means that the curvature of the penis will not get any worse. The patient no longer feels any pain except when having an erection. This is also when the chance of developing erectile dysfunction increases, along with the loss of girth and length or the softening of the end of the penis. The blood vessels surrounding the affected area are often clogged with small plaques, causing the penis to bend during an erection.

Causes

It's not always clear what causes Peyronie's Disease. However, based on patients' experiences, they are diagnosed with it because of an injury or trauma to the organ, from rough sex, sport-related accidents, and other situations that directly impact the penis. However, it is also hereditary.

During vigorous sexual intercourse, a penis may experience an injury when it is bent while penetrating or when there's pressure from the pubic bone of the partner. This kind of injury results in scar tissue formation in the penis, which contributes to Peyronie's Disease. For some reason, this process occurs outside the typical recovery pattern after an injury to the penis and results in fibrous plaques.

That said, not all men who experienced trauma on their penises get Peyronie's Disease. Some of the risk factors associated with Peyronie's Disease include:

- *Connective tissue disorder* – According to researchers, men with certain connective tissue disorders such as tympanosclerosis or scleroderma have a greater risk of getting it.
- *Age* – This disease is likely to happen as one gets older. According to statistics, at least 10-15% of middle-aged men acquire the disease.
- *Prostate cancer* – Men who have undergone prostate cancer surgery have a higher risk of getting Peyronie's Disease. This also applies to people with autoimmune disorders like lupus.

Symptoms

Aside from the described penile curvature, swelling, pain during erection, and reduced flexibility in achieving sexual pleasure with one's partner, here are some other signs to check out if you suspect you have Peyronie's Disease:

- ***Scar tissue*** – this is the formation of plaque that can be felt under the skin of the penis as a hard, flat mass.
- ***Bending of the penis*** – the curving happens upwards, downwards, or sideways depending on where the plaque forms on the penis. In some men, when the penis is erect, there are signs of narrowing or indentation on the penis.
- ***Pain*** – usually experienced whether there's an erection or not.
- ***Shortening of the penis*** – the length and girth of the organ is affected.
- ***Erectile dysfunction*** – men with Peyronie's Disease often experience difficulty getting or maintaining an erection. That said, there are cases where men report erectile dysfunction even before they show any signs of Peyronie's Disease.

That said, the curvature and length of the penis tend to worsen gradually when one has Peyronie's Disease. However, pain during erection is reported to improve within a year or two. In some cases, the penile curvature and pain associated with Peyronie's Disease tend to improve even without treatment.

There's nothing wrong with wanting to check if you have Peyronie's Disease. If you want to make sure whether you have it or not, start by observing your penis. Does it bend, curve, lose length, or girth? Do you feel plaque through its skin? When you have an erection, does your penis bend down, up, or to the side where there is scarring?

In addition to that, as you perform self-checks, you could use the following checklist to determine whether or not you are likely to have Peyronie's Disease. This way, you can better prepare to talk to a healthcare provider concerning your condition. It is no secret that sexual health and sexual function are difficult topics to discuss with anyone. This means that the more prepared you are, the easier the diagnostic process will be when you finally see a doctor. The checklist comprises answering the following questions:

- Do I experience penile pain during an erection?
- Do I have trouble getting or maintaining a firm erection as I used to?
- When I have an erection, does my penis appear curved or have an indentation or an hourglass shape? If so, has the curvature changed over time? Does the curvature pose a problem when having penetrative intercourse?
- Does my penis appear shorter than usual during an erection?
- Does my penis have plaques, lumps, nodules, or bumps?

Take note that not everyone with the disease will experience all the above symptoms. If you have one or two of these symptoms— especially if you think the disease is in your blood or you experience an accident that may have injured or caused trauma to your penis—immediately consult with your doctor to get a proper diagnosis. The good thing about early treatment is that you get a better chance of improving or preventing the condition from getting any worse.

The truth is, not all cases of Peyronie's Disease will need treatment. However, seeking immediate medical attention can go a long way in improving long-term function.

Treatment of Peyronie's Disease

According to research, at least 13 out of 100 cases of Peyronie's Disease go away without treatment. Typically, the disease is recommended to be treated without surgery, at least for the first year after diagnosis. This is especially applicable to men with small plaques, slight penile curvature, no pain, and no problems in their sexual performance.

That said, there are several treatment methods for Peyronie's Disease. Some of these include:

- **Use of oral drugs**

    This primarily targets the acute phase of Peyronie's Disease. While long-term studies have not demonstrated convincing benefits, some of the oral drugs available for treatment are:

    - ***Oral Vitamin E*** treats the plaque to minimize pain and inflammation and reduce deformity.
    - ***Tamoxifen*** is a non-steroidal anti-estrogen drug used to treat plaques.

- *Carnitine* is an antioxidant drug known to reduce swelling of the affected area of the penis, thereby promoting the healing of the wound.
- Treatment for erectile dysfunction may accompany Peyronie's Disease, such as Viagra or other oral medications to enhance blood flow through the penis, penile injections, or penile implants. In some men with severe curvature, surgery is recommended to straighten the penis.
- Exercise for men with PD to maximize flexibility, strength, blood flow, and self-image.
- Pelvic floor exercises for both men and women with Peyronie's Disease, particularly if the curvature is bothersome during intercourse or associated with voiding problems (painful urination) or bladder control (retention). Pelvic floor exercises are most effective when performed regularly.
- Counseling for psychological issues that often accompany Peyronie's Disease. Emotional distress can exacerbate physical symptoms and vice versa.

Alternative Treatments

- **Phyto-therapy**

  A research study conducted by a Turkish research group reported using a Boswellia serrata extract in the treatment of Peyronie's Disease. Research participants with Peyronie's Disease who took the plant extract significantly improved their penile curvature and plaque size. In contrast, those who took the control (placebo) had no change in their condition.

Other plant extracts that have also been used with a great improvement in penile curvature and plaque size within six months include Lawsonia inermis extract and Scutellaria lateriflora (aka blue skullcap) which has been shown to inhibit human alpha-smooth muscle actin (α-SMA), an important marker of penile fibrosis. Another study conducted in Egypt using the ginseng extract showed a significant reduction in various inflammatory markers, like TNF-alpha, IL-1 beta, and C-reactive protein (CRP) in men with this condition.

- **Extracorporeal Shockwave Therapy**

This is a non-invasive therapy that is effective in early improving erectile dysfunction.

As the name suggests, this therapy involves applying shock waves to the penis through a probe on the skin. These waves cause mild trauma to the blood vessels, stimulating the secretion of growth factors that promote the growth of new blood vessels and repair the endothelium in existing blood vessels. This creates an inflammatory reaction that triggers the breakdown of plaques within the penis, increasing blood flow, calcium reabsorption, and nerve sensitivity within the penis. The penis straightens and leads to improved sexual function and rejuvenated sexual satisfaction.

This type of therapy is safe. According to research studies, there is no evidence of long-term adverse effects of the treatment. In one study, a small percentage of research participants experienced temporary bruising in the area where the treatment was applied, but it healed in a couple of days. The only downsides to this therapy are the high cost of treatment, long time of application, and mild discomfort during treatment.

Depending on what your doctor may recommend, typically a patient will have to undergo 12 treatment sessions over six weeks. One session lasts for about 15 to 20 minutes.

- **The Platelet Rich Plasma Treatment**

  This is another natural solution that is effective in treating Peyronie's Disease. This technique harnesses growth factors in the bloodstream to stimulate the growth of new blood vessels.

  Here, blood is drawn from the patient's body and isolated growth factors. The platelet-rich plasma is then reinjected into the affected area of the penis. This stimulates an increase in the size of the penis, lowers pain, increases the frequency of erections, enhances sexual performance, stronger orgasms, and overall improvement in relationships.

Considering the biological material used is obtained from the patient's body, there are no side effects associated with this procedure.

Dealing with Peyronie's Disease

Peyronie's Disease is a condition that affects not only physically but also the patient's emotional and mental well-being. It's normal and understandable for a patient to experience having his self-confidence hurt by the effects of the disease. Additionally, dealing with this disease may prove to be challenging not only for the patient but also for his partner.

The same goes for the partner of the Peyronie's Disease patient. Both parties must understand this disease and work together to be each other's sources of support.

Schedule a doctor's appointment

Seeking medical help is a must in this situation because there are treatments available for this disease. Getting ashamed of having a problem with your penis will not help you, especially in the longer run. Best to seek help as soon as possible, even if you only need to make sure you don't have it.

You were probably in an accident a while back, and while you didn't feel any pain or trauma from it, it's still better to have it ruled out than suffer the consequences later.

Talk to someone you trust

One best way to deal with it after getting diagnosed is to talk about it to someone you trust. It may be your partner, a friend, or even your father. This way, someone will be able to look after you and be your source of support, especially during treatments. Choose to talk to someone who you know will take the time to understand your situation. It's also important that you know you can trust them so you will be at ease mentally.

Involve your partner

Having open lines of honest communication with your partner goes a long way in helping you feel more comfortable about the condition and how it impacts your sex life. Talk to your partner about any pain or discomfort you might be experiencing during intercourse. By letting them in on your concerns, you are allowing them a chance to offer you support, eliminate misunderstandings and preserve your relationship.

While dealing with Peyronie's Disease is difficult for you, you must understand that it is difficult for your partner as well. If not handled well, it can seriously impact your self-image and relationship. Various studies have linked the disease to decreased self-esteem issues, depression, and loss of sexual confidence. As a partner to someone with Peyronie's Disease, you realize that your partner needs help, support, and treatment.

Remember that you are not alone

Another important thing to remember is that you are not an isolated case. Nearly 10% of men have this condition, and most tend to feel isolated. This shouldn't have to be the case.

If your partner has this, let them know that you understand and are willing to walk with them every step of the way. Let them know that there are several sources of information about the condition and treatment. Give them suggestions of websites or sources of this information. Discuss with him the possibility of having normal erections. The last thing you want to do is make them feel less masculine, which tends to be magnified in men with Peyronie's Disease. Understand that most men are embarrassed by their condition, which might make them feel uncomfortable talking to you or anyone else about it.

Create a safe space in your relationship

Considering this condition affects both of you, make the conversation as comfortable as possible. At first, he might be resistant, but starting the discussion is the first step toward seeking treatment. Explain to him how you feel about his condition and how it impacts your relationship. Let him know that you want to help. Be gentle and soft about it. You could say something like, "Honey, our sex life has been enjoyable and is an important part of our overall relationship. In light of your condition, I would like to help to continue enjoying intimacy. I have read online, and different treatments can help. Let's book an appointment with the doctor to know more."

The key here is to be as supportive as possible. Pay attention to how he feels. Quit making assumptions about him because that will only make matters worse. You want them to feel that you care about them. In the meantime, you can also explore non-sexual intimacy options like cuddling, holding hands, massages, and kissing to stay physically connected and make it easier to walk this path together.

The Connection Between Diet and Peyronie's Disease

While there has not been any scientific evidence of how diet could cause, worsen, cure, or treat Peyronie's Disease, a good diet could still potentially help mitigate or manage this condition.

The more you eat a healthy and balanced diet, the better your body is equipped to deal with physical trauma, whether it is Peyronie's Disease or other health issues.

A good healthy diet plays an important role in improving overall health and boosting the immune system. This way, the body can heal from traumas like Peyronie's Disease. Hence the reason you must consider incorporating healthy food choices into your diet.

What would your diet plan entail?

It should have fresh, unprocessed, unrefined foods. These include:

Fruits like apples, blueberries, avocados, oranges, and watermelon.

- Eggs
- Fish – e.g., salmon, albacore tuna, trout, herring, swordfish, sardines, and mackerel.
- Milk and dairy products like
- Pulses like beans, nuts – e.g., Almonds and Walnuts – and seeds – e.g., pistachios
- Starchy foods, like whole bread, rice, pasta, and potatoes.
- Vegetables like spinach, leafy greens, tomatoes, and peppers.
- White meat like chicken

That said, there are several foods you should avoid. These include:

- Coffee
- Carbonated and energy drinks
- Alcohol
- Refined and processed foods
- White bread

Implementing Your Diet Plan

Now that you know what you should eat and avoid, how do you implement the diet plan?

By incorporating a healthy eating plan into your everyday lifestyle. At first, it is easy to feel discouraged, but with just a few instructions and modifications to your daily habits, you will be on your way to a healthy lifestyle for the long haul.

Step 1: Decide which meal planning style suits you

What meals are you going to cook and eat for the week? Use that to create a grocery list. The key here is to choose a meal-planning style that works best for you. You must set up a healthy waiting environment. Get your family together at mealtimes and enjoy food together rather than spending meal times in front of a time, leading to mindless eating.

Step 2: Stock up your pantry

For your meal planning to be easier and less intimidating, it is necessary always to stock up your pantry. Select recipes that will support your health and then use them to create a list of groceries to buy before going out for grocery shopping.

Additionally, ensure that your kitchen has the necessary equipment for cooking and storing meals – knives, pans, storage containers, and storage bags.

Once you have your list, the next thing is to schedule a day to go shopping. For most people, it is easier to plan on Saturday and then go out shopping on Sunday. The key is to find a day that works best for you and then be consistent for meal planning to be part of your weekly routine.

That said, your meal plans are not cast in stone. You must stay flexible to accommodate days when unpredictable events happen or don't have the time or energy to stick to the plan.

Step 3: Incorporate your plan into your social activities

It is hard not to find food whenever you socialize with people. That does not mean you should sacrifice healthy foods for the sake of fitting in. If there are gatherings, plan to bring healthy foods ahead of time instead of indulging in barbecues slathered with processed sauces and saturated fats. Go for healthy potlucks featuring whole foods, veggies, and fruits if you are hosting.

The other trick is to engage in activities that don't necessarily have food as the primary focus. While most people use food as a way to soothe the heart, fend off boredom, celebrate, or socialize, you can choose to create a new culture for yourself. Realize that when food becomes the center of focus, it can be challenging to stick to a healthy eating plan. Therefore, choose to go hiking, biking, painting, or even gardening as a form of socializing.

Step 4: Learn to read nutrition labels

When making healthier eating choices, you must pay attention to the nutrition facts labels. This way, you can easily identify and pick out nutrient-dense and healthy foods.

What should you look for in labels?

- Look at the serving information to know the size a single serving has; and the total number of servings in each package.
- Consider the calories per serving and in each package. Understand that the moment you double your serving, you double the calories and nutrients as well. You must learn to limit certain nutrients such as added sugars, sodium, and saturated fats. You should also avoid anything that contains trans fats. The key is to go for a package loaded with enough beneficial nutrients like calcium, dietary fiber, potassium, choline, iron, and Vitamins A, C, D, and E.

Step 5: Get rid of certain foods and bad habits

Take a minute to think about your eating habits—are they good or bad?

It doesn't matter whether you have had the same eating habits for years, the good news is that it is never too late to adjust. While sudden and radical changes may seem like a good idea at first, it is not healthy and may not be sustainable in the long run.

To improve your eating habits permanently, you need an intentional approach that requires you to:

Reflect

- Start by creating a list of all your eating and drinking habits
- Highlight the habits on your list that may lead to unhealthy choices
- Pay attention to the habits you just highlighted and try to find their triggers
- Now, ask yourself whether there is something you can do to avoid the trigger or things you can do differently to be healthier

Replace

Now, start replacing the unhealthy habits with healthy choices like dropping foods with trans fats, eating only when hungry, and planning meals to ensure you only eat a healthy, well-balanced diet.

Reinforce

Now that you have learned new, healthy habits to replace the old unhealthy habits, the most important thing is to reinforce them. Realize that habits take time to develop. This will not happen overnight, hence the need to exercise patience. Beware of the things you put into your body and make changes as soon as you notice anything out of place. One step at a time, and you will be a healthy version of yourself. So, keep going—you can do it!

Step 6: Leverage easy meal prep tips

Remember, making healthy choices is not magic – it will not happen overnight. The most important thing is to start small and then slowly build your confidence to ensure the sustainability of new habits. For instance, you can start by planning out a few meals for a day and slowly work towards a week.

As you do this, you must consider each food group and emphasize whole foods such as whole grains, veggies, fruits, healthy fats, legumes, and high-quality proteins. Limit your added sugars, refined and processed foods, and excess salt.

You must also pay attention to your kitchen, pantry, and refrigerator organization. The more organized you get, the more successful your meal plans are. Consistently carve out time—say 10-15 minutes every week— to craft a meal plan. Set aside a place in the kitchen to store your recipes, digital or written format, to avoid any frustrations and make referencing easy during cooking.

It is also advisable to always buy in bulk. This way, you stock up your pantry with healthy foods and save time, money and reduce any unnecessary packaging waste.

Finally, make your meal prep enjoyable. Quit thinking of it as something you have to do and instead consider it a form of self-care. Make your meal preps a family affair by involving your partner and children. While this might seem overwhelming at first because of all the changes, you can leverage different strategies to develop sustainable meal-planning habits that suit your lifestyle.

Sample Recipes

Garlic Hummus

Ingredients:

- 12 heads of garlic, roasted
- 2 tsp. virgin coconut oil
- 2 12-cup muffin tins
- extra trays of ice cube

Instructions:

1. Preheat the oven to 400°F.
2. Cut off the top of each garlic head to make the top of the cloves visible.
3. Put each garlic head in a muffin tin cup.
4. Rub the top of the garlic heads with coconut oil.
5. Use the second muffin tin to cover the first one.
6. Put in the oven and wait for 30 minutes to bake.
7. Take the garlic cloves out of the heads.
8. You may place 4-5 cloves of garlic in each ice cube tray section to store leftovers.
9. Use olive oil to cover cloves and freeze.
10. Squeeze the frozen roasted garlic cubes out of the trays and store them using a container.

Salmon and Asparagus

Ingredients:

- 2 salmon filets
- 14-oz. young potatoes
- 8 asparagus spears, trimmed and halved
- 2 handfuls cherry tomatoes
- 1 handful basil leaves
- 2 tbsp. extra-virgin olive oil
- 1 tbsp. balsamic vinegar

Instructions:

1. Heat oven to 428°F.
2. Arrange potatoes into a baking dish.
3. Drizzle potatoes with extra-virgin olive oil.
4. Roast potatoes until they have turned golden brown.
5. Place asparagus into the baking dish together with the potatoes.
6. Roast in the oven for 15 minutes.
7. Arrange cherry tomatoes and salmon among the vegetables.
8. Drizzle with balsamic vinegar and the remaining olive oil.
9. Roast until the salmon is cooked.
10. Throw in basil leaves before transferring everything to a serving dish.
11. Serve while hot.

Tahini Salmon

Instructions:

- 1/4 cup tahini
- 3 tbsp. fresh lemon juice
- 1 tsp. mashed garlic
- 1/4 tsp. salt
- 1/2 cup finely chopped cilantro
- 2 tbsp. roughly chopped toasted walnuts
- 2 tbsp. roughly chopped toasted almonds
- 1 tbsp. finely chopped onion
- 1 tsp. extra-virgin olive oil
- cayenne
- black pepper, freshly ground
- 1 lb. wild salmon skin removed, fresh or frozen

Instructions:

1. In a bowl, combine the tahini, 2 tbsp. of lemon juice, 3 tbsp. of water, mashed garlic, and 1/8 tsp. of salt; set aside
2. In a separate bowl, combine the cilantro, walnuts, almonds, onion, olive oil, cayenne, black pepper, and 1/8 tsp. of salt.
3. Fill the bottom of a steamer with water and bring it to a boil.
4. Season fish with 1 tbsp. of lemon juice.

5. Place it on a plate and put it on top of the steamer. Cover and cook, taking care to remove while the fish is still pink inside, about 3 to 4 minutes.
6. Remove the fish from the steamer, top with the tahini mixture, and then with the cilantro mixture.
7. Serve warm or at room temperature.

Salmon with Avocados and Brussels Sprouts

Ingredients:

- 2 lbs. of salmon filet, divided into 4 pieces
- 1 tsp. ground cumin
- 1 tsp. onion powder
- 1 tsp. paprika powder
- 1/2 tsp. garlic powder
- 1 tsp. chili powder
- Himalayan sea salt
- black pepper, freshly ground

Avocado sauce:

- 2 chopped avocados
- 1 lime, squeezed for the juice
- 1 tbsp. extra-virgin olive oil
- 1 tbsp. fresh minced cilantro
- 1 diced small red onion
- 1 minced garlic clove
- Himalayan sea salt to taste
- black pepper, freshly ground

Brussels sprouts:

- 3 lbs. of Brussels sprouts
- 1/2 cup raw honey
- 1/2 cup balsamic vinegar
- 1/2 cup melted coconut oil

- 1 cup dried cranberries
- Himalayan sea salt
- black pepper, freshly ground

Instructions:

To make the salmon and avocado sauce:

1. Combine cumin, onion, chili powder, garlic, and paprika seasoned with salt and pepper. Mix well before dry rubbing on the salmon.
2. Place the salmon in the fridge for 30 minutes.
3. Preheat the grill.
4. In a bowl, mash avocado until the texture becomes smooth. Pour in all the remaining ingredients and mix thoroughly.
5. Grill salmon for 5 minutes on each side or until cooked.
6. Drizzle avocado on cooked salmon.

To prepare the Brussels sprouts:

1. Preheat the oven to 375°F.
2. Mix Brussels sprouts with coconut oil. Season with salt and pepper.
3. Place vegetables on a baking sheet and roast for about 30 minutes.
4. In a separate pan, combine vinegar and honey.
5. Simmer in slow heat until it boils and thickens.
6. Drizzle them on top of the Brussels sprouts.

7. Serve with the salmon.

Chicken Breast Delight

Ingredients:

- 1 tsp. dried oregano
- 1/2 tsp. rosemary
- 1/2 tsp. garlic powder
- 1/8 tsp. salt
- finely ground black pepper
- 4 chicken breasts

Instructions:

1. Remove any fat from the breasts.
2. Mix the remaining ingredients in a separate container.
3. Add the mixture to either side of the chicken.
4. Prepare a frying pan, lightly oil the pan, and set the stove to medium.
5. Add the chicken to the frying pan. Cook for 3 to 5 minutes on each face.
6. Cool the chicken for a couple of minutes after cooking.
7. Serve warm.

Steak with Olive Oil

Ingredients:

- 2 8-oz. grass-fed New York strip steaks, about 1-1/2-inch-thick, trimmed
- 3 tbsp. olive oil, divided
- 1 tsp. freshly ground black pepper, divided
- 1 tsp. kosher salt, divided
- 1 garlic clove, crushed
- 1 rosemary sprig
- optional: rosemary leaves

Instructions:

1. Place the grill pan over medium-high heat.
2. Brush a tablespoon of oil on the steak, then sprinkle with half a teaspoon of salt and another half teaspoon of pepper.
3. Put a tablespoon of oil into the pan, followed by a rosemary sprig and garlic.
4. Cook steak for about 9 minutes, or until preferred doneness is achieved. For every minute, turn the steak and baste it with oil.
5. Transfer the steak to a cutting board, letting it rest for 5 minutes.

6. Slice steak across the grain and place it on a platter. Drizzle with the juice from the cutting board and the leftover oil.
7. Sprinkle it with the remaining salt and pepper.
8. Upon serving, garnish with rosemary leaves if desired.

Garlic Broccoli Salad

Ingredients:

- 1 head broccoli, cut into florets
- 1 tsp. olive oil
- 1-1/2 tbsp. rice wine vinegar
- 1 tbsp. sesame oil
- 2 cloves garlic, minced
- 1 pinch cayenne pepper
- 3 tbsp. golden raisins

Instructions:

1. Fill water into a steamer. Bring to a boil.
2. Add broccoli. Cover. Steam until tender for about 3 minutes.
3. Rinse broccoli and set aside.
4. Heat olive oil in a skillet over medium heat.
5. Put in pine nuts. Stir fry for 1-2 minutes.
6. Remove from heat.
7. Whisk together rice vinegar, sesame oil, pepper, and garlic.
8. Transfer the broccoli, nuts, and raisins to the rice vinegar dressing.
9. Serve and enjoy.

Mixed Vegetable Roast with Lemon Zest

Ingredients:

- 1-1/2 cups broccoli florets
- 1-1/2 cups cauliflower florets
- 3/4 cup red bell pepper, diced
- 3/4 cup zucchini, diced
- 2 thinly sliced cloves of garlic
- 2 tsp. lemon zest
- 1 tbsp. olive oil
- a pinch of salt
- 1 tsp. dried and crushed oregano

Instructions:

1. Preheat the oven at 425°F for 25 minutes.
2. Combine garlic and florets of broccoli and cauliflower in a baking pan.
3. Drizzle oil evenly over the vegetables. Season with salt and oregano.
4. Stir the vegetables to coat them evenly.
5. Place the pan inside the oven and roast for 10 minutes.
6. Add zucchini and bell pepper to the mix. Toss to combine.
7. Continue roasting for 10 to 15 minutes more until the vegetables turn light brown.
8. Drizzle lemon zest over vegetables and toss.
9. Serve and enjoy.

Spinach and Watercress Salad

Ingredients:

- 1 cup watercress, washed with stems removed
- 3 cups baby spinach, washed with stems removed
- 1 medium sliced avocado
- 1/4 cup avocado oil
- 1/8 cup lemon juice
- a pinch of salt

Instructions:

1. Pat dry the spinach and watercress. Remove the stem and separate the leaves.
2. On a large serving plate, combine the leaves of the watercress and the spinach.
3. Cut the avocado in half, then remove the pit. Peel the skin off from each side.
4. Slice the avocados into thin strips. Set aside.
5. Prepare the dressing by combining avocado oil and lemon juice.
6. Arrange the avocado strips on top of the watercress and spinach.
7. Season with salt and pepper.

Vegetable Broth

Ingredients:

- 1 tbsp. oil
- 2 leeks, sliced
- 2 carrots, sliced
- 2 ribs celery
- 1/4 tsp. salt
- 8 cups water

To make the soup:

- 1 tbsp. oil
- 2 cups potatoes, diced
- 1 cup mushrooms, diced
- 1-1/2 cups cauliflower, diced
- 1 cup onion, diced
- 1 cup celery, diced
- 1 cup carrot, diced
- 1-1/2 cups red beans, cooked
- 2 sprigs rosemary
- 4 sprigs thyme
- 2 cups spinach

Instructions:

1. To a pot on medium heat, add oil and leeks.
2. Cook for about three minutes or until they start to soften up.

3. Add carrots and top a few celery stalks with leaves.
4. Cover with water.
5. Add salt. Bring to a simmer and cook until carrots are very tender but not mushy.
6. Turn off the heat and let it cool down a little.
7. When the broth has cooled down, strain out the veggies.
8. Remove carrots and set them aside.
9. Squeeze most of the liquid out of the leeks and celery.

To cook the soup:

1. Add carrots to some of the broth and blend.
2. With a pot on medium heat, add oil, onions, raw carrots, and celery. Cook until onions are translucent, approximately 3 to 5 minutes.
3. Add broth, potatoes, and herbs.
4. Bring to a simmer and cook for 10 minutes.
5. Add cauliflower and red beans.
6. Simmer for another 5 minutes.
7. Add the package of frozen green beans and cook until the potatoes and cauliflower are tender, approximately for another 5 minutes.
8. At the end of cooking, add spinach.
9. Serve warm.

Salad Medley

Ingredients:

- 4 artichokes, halved
- 1/2 avocado, sliced into thin wedges
- 1/2 red, yellow, or green bell pepper, thinly sliced
- 1/4 squash, thinly sliced
- 1/2 zucchini, thinly sliced
- 1/2 red, yellow, or green onion, thinly sliced
- 1 cup mushrooms, thinly sliced
- 1 cup broccoli
- 1/4 cup broccoli sprouts
- 1 cup cauliflower
- 1 cup spinach
- 1 cup kale
- 1 bunch leeks, chopped
- 1/4 cup raw sunflower seeds, sprouted
- 1/4 cup raw almonds, sprouted
- 1/4 cup garbanzo beans, sprouted
- 1/4 cup mung beans, sprouted
- 1/4 cup red or green lentils, sprouted
- 1/4 cup purple cabbage, shredded
- 2 tbsp. extra-virgin olive oil

Instructions:

1. Steam vegetables in a saucepan with 1-inch water for 5 to 10 minutes.

2. Transfer steamed vegetables into a serving bowl.
3. Drizzle with extra-virgin olive oil.
4. Toss the vegetables.
5. Serve immediately.

Quinoa Lentil Salad

Ingredients:

- 2/3 cups dried brown lentils
- 2 cups water
- 1 cup quinoa
- 1 yellow sweet pepper, diced
- 1 shallot, chopped
- 1 bunch arugula, finely chopped
- 2 tsp. Dijon mustard
- 1/4 cup lemon juice
- 1/4 cup extra virgin olive oil
- 1/3 cup crumbled feta cheese
- 1 pinch salt
- 4 tbsp. fresh mint, chopped

Instructions:

1. Bring 2 cups of salt water to a boil in a saucepan.
2. Toss veggies into boiling salt water. Lower heat, and cook for 30 minutes.
3. Drain lentils and discard water. Set veggies aside.
4. Boil another batch of saltwater, and cook the quinoa in the pan.

5. In a bowl, mix pepper, salt, mustard, lemon juice, and oil.
6. Place veggies in a larger bowl, and pour the mixture.
7. Sprinkle mint and feta cheese over the salad.
8. Serve and enjoy.

Fruit and Dark Greens Salad

Ingredients:

- 1 cup watermelon
- 1 cup cucumber sliced or spiral
- 1/2 cup raspberries
- 1 sliced avocado
- 1 cup baby broccoli
- 1 cup papaya
- 1/2 cup toasted almonds
- 4 cups baby kale

Dressing:

- 1/2 cup olive oil
- 1/2 cup master tonic
- 1/4 cup goji berries
- 4 dates
- a pinch of sea salt

Tonic:

- 1/4 cup garlic, minced
- 1/4 cup onion, chopped
- 2 tbsp. horseradish, minced
- 2 knobs turmeric, chopped
- 1 jalapeno pepper, chopped
- 32 oz. organic apple cider vinegar
- 1/4 cup fresh ginger, chopped

- juice of 1 lemon

Instructions:
1. Mix all salad ingredients except almonds.
2. Toss salad.

To make the dressing:
1. Mix master tonic, olive oil, and salt together.
2. In a blender, blend goji berries and dates until smooth.
3. Upon serving the salad, drizzle the dressing on, and gently add almonds.

To make the master tonic:
1. Add all ingredients to apple cider vinegar.
2. Blend all ingredients until everything is mixed well.
3. Let the tonic sit in a jar for 1 to 2 weeks, shaking periodically.
4. Strain first before adding the leftover vinegar mixture into a jar with a cover.

Conclusion

Thank you again for getting this guide.

If you found this guide helpful, please take the time to share your thoughts and post a review. It'd be greatly appreciated!

Thank you and good luck!

References and Helpful Links

Alkandari, M. H., Touma, N., & Carrier, S. (2021). Platelet-Rich Plasma Injections for Erectile Dysfunction and Peyronie's Disease: A Systematic Review of Evidence. Sexual medicine reviews.

Bagchi, M., Patel, S., Zafra-Stone, S., & Bagchi, D. (2011). Selected herbal supplements and nutraceuticals. In Reproductive and Developmental Toxicology (pp. 385-393). Academic Press.

Bjekic, M. D., Vlajinac, H. D., Sipetic, S. B., & Marinkovic, J. M. (2006). Risk factors for Peyronie's Disease: A case-control study. BJU international, 97(3), 570-574.

Chatzichristodoulou, G., Meisner, C., Gschwend, J. E., Stenzl, A., & Lahme, S. (2013). Extracorporeal shock wave therapy in Peyronie's Disease: Results of a placebo-controlled, prospective, randomized, single-blind study. The journal of sexual medicine, 10(11), 2815-2821.

Epifanova, M. V., Gvasalia, B. R., Durashov, M. A., & Artemenko, S. A. (2020). Platelet-rich plasma therapy for male sexual dysfunction: myth or reality?. Sexual Medicine Reviews, 8(1), 106-113.

Gelbard, M. K., Dorey, F., & James, K. (1990). The natural history of Peyronie's Disease. The Journal of Urology, 144(6), 1376-1379.

Gholami, S. S., Gonzalez-Cadavid, N. F., Lin, C. S., Rajfer, J., & Lue, T. F. (2003). Peyronie's Disease: a review. The Journal of Urology, 169(4), 1234-1241.

Nehra, A., Alterowitz, R., Culkin, D. J., Faraday, M. M., Hakim, L. S., Heidelbaugh, J. J., ... & Burnett, A. L. (2015). Peyronie's Disease: AUA guideline. The Journal of Urology, 194(3), 745-753.

"Peyronie's Disease." Peyronie's Disease: Symptoms, Diagnosis & Treatment - Urology Care Foundation. Accessed February 19, 2022. https://www.urologyhealth.org/urology-a-z/p/peyronies-disease.

Srirangam, S. J., Manikandan, R., Hussain, J., Collins, G. N., & O'Reilly, P. H. (2006). Long-term results of extracorporeal shockwave therapy for Peyronie's Disease. Journal of endourology, 20(11), 880-884.

Yarnell, E., & Abascal, K. (2013). Antifibrotic herbs: indications, mechanisms of action, doses, and safety information. Alternative and Complementary Therapies, 19(2), 75-82.

www.ingramcontent.com/pod-product-compliance
Lightning Source LLC
LaVergne TN
LVHW012038060526
838201LV00061B/4666